Dr. Earl Mindell's

What You Should Know About Trace Minerals

Dr. Earl Mindell's

What You Should Know About Trace Minerals

Earl L. Mindell, R.Ph., Ph.D.

with Virginia L. Hopkins

Dr. Earl Mindell's What You Should Know About Trace Minerals is intended solely for informational and educational purposes, and not as medical advice. Please consult a medical or health professional if you have questions about your health.

Printed in the United States of America

Book Margins, Inc.
A BMI Edition

By arrangement with Keats Publishing, Inc.

We would like to thank Maria Gordon
for her expert assistance
in writing and researching this book.

Contents

CHAPTER 1

The Role of Trace Minerals

Everyone has heard of the essential minerals calcium and magnesium, but relatively few know of the importance of the trace minerals, such as chromium, vanadium and selenium. Although the trace minerals comprise less than four percent of our total body weight, their presence, absence or imbalance can mean the difference between health and illness, and even between life and death.

Vitamins cannot function without trace minerals. Trace minerals also play a role in regulating hormones, enzymes, amino acids and the immune system. They are required to build and maintain the structure of the body, and to maintain proper brain function, blood sugar balance and to keep the intestines healthy and fully functioning. In other words, trace minerals are involved in every aspect of health and balance in the human body. While the body can synthesize some vitamins, it cannot manufacture a single trace mineral, and can withstand a deficiency of vitamins longer than a deficiency of minerals. In turn, vitamins play a role in the uptake and utilization of trace minerals.

Although trace mineral consumption is tiny compared to that of energy-providing foods, they perform fundamental chemical tasks in an extremely wide range of vital animal and plant functions. The quantities of minerals required are no measure of their importance in the human body. While many so-called major minerals such as calcium and magnesium are needed in milligram amounts, most trace minerals are needed in microgram amounts!

The minute amounts of trace minerals needed have meant their importance was largely undiscovered until the 20th century. Once uncovered, however, the activity of trace minerals opened a giant chest of subtle but very powerful tools for fine-tuning the body for optimal health, increasing the benefits of exercise, and even preventing cancer, heart disease and diabetes. Learn about trace minerals and you will have found a way to fine-tune your personal nutrition to maximize your health.

THE STORY OF MINERALS

The story of minerals is as old as the earth, with billions of years of participation in the very formation of life on this planet. Before animal and vegetable, there was mineral in the form of chemical elements such as iron and silicon. Primeval rains created the first oceans and washed minerals into the seas, quickening the pace of evolution in the first chapter of life.

The sciences of biochemistry, physics and geology continue to unravel the mysteries of the minerals needed for life. I found a *New York Times* story about sulfur of particular interest: According to this article, some researchers believe the asteroid collision thought to have led to the extinction of the dinosaurs resulted in wide distribution of the trace element sulfur. The asteroid was especially rich in sulfur and is thought to have vaporized, creating more than 100 billion tons of mainly sulfur dioxide in the atmosphere, increasing the availability of sulfur for the life forms that evolved after the dinosaurs.

WHAT ARE MINERALS?

To be technical, minerals are inorganic chemical elements. Inorganic means not bound to carbon. Sometimes minerals are described as inorganic when they have not been dissolved in water or transformed by plants. "Inorganic" minerals are harder for the body to absorb than those in organic form. While the chemical structure of the minerals themselves doesn't change, they may be attached to other molecules that give them different properties.

Since the origin of multicellular life minerals have been important for their ability to bond to themselves and other substances in animals and plants. In this way they help create important chemical compounds. The trace mineral cobalt is a component of vitamin B12, and iron is a part of hemoglobin. The total of about 22 dietary minerals are needed for optimal human health.

Rocks remain the original source of minerals, since living matter cannot synthesize them as it can most vitamins. Fortunately, we don't have to serve up pebbles and stones with meals! Nature has instead provided pathways for minerals, taking them from soil and water to plants and animals. Wise eating, drinking and use of supplements insures that we take in just enough dietary minerals to keep our bodies fully functional.

WHAT ARE TRACE MINERALS?

In a 150-pound body, some two to three pounds is the mineral calcium, which we need to get from what we eat. Vanadium, in contrast, would be difficult even to measure, and yet it is a trace mineral that can help reverse adult-onset diabetes in the form of the compound vanadyl sulfate.

The definition of what exactly a trace mineral is varies, but in general it is a mineral that makes up less than 0.01 percent of body weight. The major minerals, or macrominerals, each make up more than 0.01 percent of body weight. Although a few trace minerals such as zinc are needed in milligram amounts daily, most are needed in only microgram amounts. Trace minerals are sometimes called "trace elements," and those needed to maintain health are called "essential" trace minerals or elements.

The macrominerals essential to human health are calcium, phosphorus, magnesium, potassium, sodium and chloride. The trace minerals we will cover in some detail in this book, either because they are essential to optimal health or because they can play a key role in healing, are boron, chromium, cobalt, copper, fluorine, iodine, iron, lithium, manganese, molybdenum, selenium, vanadium and zinc. Trace minerals that are found in the body but which are poisonous in very small amounts when inhaled, absorbed or ingested include arsenic, aluminum, cadmium, lead, mercury, nickel and tin. Toxicity caused by these metals is largely a result of by-products of manufacturing and pollution.

The tiniest amounts of trace minerals are all that is needed to keep body functions running smoothly, but a deficiency has quite obvious effects. For example, in the absence of only a little over one millionth of an ounce of iodine, the thyroid gland enlarges.

The nutritional role of copper and iron may have been unknown in ancient times, but along with other minerals, they were believed to possess spiritual powers. Although the story of essential trace minerals and humans began hundreds of thousands of years ago, it remained mostly untold until the 20th century. In 1928 just three trace elements were recognized: Iron, which was found in the 17th century to be needed for healthy blood; iodine, shown in 1850 to prevent goiter (thyroid deficiency); and copper, found in 1928 to be needed for the absorption and utilization of iron. In the ensuing decades, other trace minerals were found to play a role in maintaining health. It wasn't until the '80s that boron and vanadium were added to the list of important trace minerals.

WHERE ARE TRACE MINERALS FOUND?

Trace minerals are washed from rocks into streams and lakes, and they are naturally found in food. Tiny mineral particles also form layers of subsoil and are absorbed by water passing by or through. Plants need minerals to function and have evolved methods for absorbing them efficiently from soil and water. In turn, animals meet most of their mineral needs by eating plants. Humans meet their minerals needs by eating both plants and animals, and drinking water. The cycle continues as man, animals and plants die, eventually returning their mineral content to the environment.

It is impossible to specify the quantities of any trace mineral likely to be found in foods. Soil conditions, time of year, weather, and environmental pollution all influence mineral levels. The way a trace mineral is chemically packaged within a food is as important as its quantity. Different mineral compounds are absorbed more or less easily during digestion. Spinach, for example, has traditionally been considered a rich source of iron. In fact, it contains iron oxalate, which makes the iron only partially available to the human body. Parsley offers a form of iron that is much easier for the body to assimilate.

Knowing which foods are typically high in a particular trace mineral is useful when it comes to planning a healthy diet. Just one Brazil nut (find an unshelled, organically grown one if possible) a day, for example, can provide a daily dose of selenium. However, it remains important to eat a variety of foods to increase the number of sources and varieties of trace minerals in the diet.

CHAPTER 2

Trace Minerals and Health

Copper, iron, manganese and zinc are trace minerals needed by all bacteria, algae, fungi and higher plants for survival. Boron is required by green plants and algae, while some also need cobalt and molybdenum. This has been true for billions of years, since the first primitive organisms in the world's oceans began to develop. As life evolved, relatively advanced chemical structures were created, with minerals as major components. One such structure was chlorophyll, the substance in plants which uses the energy of light to convert carbon dioxide and water to carbohydrates. At the center of chlorophyll is the major mineral magnesium. In this way, the same silver-white flaring metal used in flashbulbs and fireworks is crucial to any vegetable or part of a grazing animal you might eat.

The trace mineral molybdenum is used by blue-green algae and other plant life to turn nitrogen into a usable compound essential to all life. Wherever we turn, minerals are in action contributing to processes that are key to life on earth.

In humans, trace minerals are involved in protein, hormone and vitamin formation; immunity, muscle function, and nerve transmission. Zinc, for example, is used in practically every cell process. The strong, consistent structure of minerals makes them essential in the body's structures, from the calcium, phosphorus and boron in the bones to silicon, which is an important component of collagen, the principal structural component found in skin. Silicon forms long, complex molecules, suitable for parts of the body, like skin, that need to be strong and flexible. Vitamin C is another major component of collagen.

Minerals are well known for their role as catalysts, speeding up chemical reactions in the body. Catalysts help the formation or breakdown of substances to occur with less energy than the original chemicals involved would need on their own. Needing less energy, life processes such as digestion and healing can occur more quickly and efficiently. Without catalysts, many essential biological reactions would take place too slowly to sustain life. Throughout any reaction, in a very neat arrangement, catalysts themselves remain unchanged, ready for re-use. The trace mineral molybdenum, for example, activates an enzyme (another type of catalyst) which detoxifies harmful preservative compounds called sulfites.

You could say that minerals act as wheelbarrows, forklifts, gears, conveyor belts and electronic switches in the factory of the body, assisting at every step from unloading the fuel trucks and stoking and damping the boilers to switching the wiring and oiling the machinery.

The importance of all this work? Tachycardia—rapid heartbeat—can be caused by a lack of potassium; diabetes can be brought on by a shortage of chromium and zinc; anemia can be caused by a lack of iron through a deficiency of cobalt, which is also required in vitamin B12 and is needed for the absorption of iron.

Prevention of disease through adequate mineral uptake should be a natural result of our nutritional intake. The increasing pollution, intensive farming, deforestation, food refining and use of medical drugs during the 20th century, however, have depleted dietary minerals and increased our exposure to minerals that are toxic in small amounts. The need is greater than ever before to ensure an adequate mineral supply for anyone interested in maintaining good health.

THE ELECTROLYTE POWER OF MINERALS

The best minerals come shaken, not stirred! Minerals are at their most powerful in forms which conduct electricity. Electrically charged minerals are known as "ionized salts" or electrolytes. Electrolytes are produced naturally as minerals are swept up and tumbled by water rushing past rocks. Homeopathic medicines, often diluted forms of minerals, are produced by deliberately simulating this natural process through vigorous shaking. The electrical charge of electrolytes makes them valuable triggers of processes in cells. Ionized mineral particles are small enough to pass directly through cell walls, bypassing the digestive process, to be absorbed within minutes of being taken. In this way minerals can act as a charge to cells which, in turn are like batteries supplying energy to the body.

Solutions of ionized minerals are described as "crystalloid." Crystalloid solutions increase the availability of minerals to the body. Minerals also exist in more inert forms as part of "colloid" suspensions. Colloid is the term used for fairly large particles unable to dissolve but able to remain partially suspended in water. Minerals in colloidal form do not pass through animal and plant membranes as easily as electrolytes in crystalloid solutions. "The best of both worlds would be to microencapsulate ionized and colloidal minerals in soy phosphatide microspheres for optimum absorption through the transmucosal membranes of the mouth. This allows for rapid sublingual absorption and bypasses the harsh digestive system."

Soil and plants in good condition contain all the

ingredients necessary to ionize colloidal minerals, preparing them for absorption. Similarly, a healthy diet ensures a nutritionally balanced body that is adapted to absorb minerals. Hydrochloric acid softens minerals, making sure, with the help of vitamins, that they travel from the gut and into the bloodstream. Once in the bloodstream, vitamins and other substances help to ionize minerals as necessary which enables them to move into the tissues of the body where they are required.

Mineral supplements become necessary because modern farming, irrigation, pollution and water cleansing have produced food and water supplies robbed of electrolytes. Food produced using modern methods may be cheaper, but it is also a nutritional rip-off. Buy organic as much as you can and rest assured the extra dollars are harnessing valuable electrolyte power.

CHAPTER 3

How Minerals Are Depleted

Evolution has led to a system in which minerals move from soil and water to plants, animals and humans. Sustainability marks the beauty of the system as minerals return intact to soil and water through the rot and decay of organic matter. Until the industrial revolution of the 19th century, the cycle of minerals was mainly undisturbed and vegetables, meat, fish and dairy foods were reliable sources of most minerals.

Ironically, as science continues to reveal more and more about the value of minerals, they have become less and less easily available from food. The story behind this unhappy scenario is largely one of refined foods, medical drugs, chemical fertilizers, pollution and deforestation. The mineral depletion so evident in today's crop-growing soils and fast foods is reflected in the depleted state of health of people all over the world, with escalating rates of killer illnesses like cancer and heart disease.

Bringing our individual mineral intakes up to par is an important dietary action. It's also worth remembering that our own actions as consumers, workers, drivers and gardeners are influencing the mineral levels of the world we live in.

SOIL LOSS IS MINERAL LOSS

The mineral-rich result of 100 to 1,000 years of natural processes is one inch of topsoil rich in minerals and other nutrients. An unprotected layer of soil ten times this thick can disappear in the trail of a bulldozer or the puff of a violent storm. Environmentally unsound farming practices and the paving of civilization have led to a steady depletion of a precious natural resource the world over.

According to Bernard Jensen and Mark Anderson in the important book *Empty Harvest* (Avery Publishing, 1990), when pioneers first crossed North America they settled on land with topsoils 18 to 25 inches deep. Today, the figure in most states is around six inches, often less. Out of the total measurement of soil erosion in the U.S., 90 percent occurs on farmland. Midwestern states like Wyoming and Nebraska have literally seen their soils blown away creating huge "dust bowls" where farmers once led a prosperous life. The days of the farming disasters of the Great Plains are still with us. North Dakota lost 3.5 million acres of topsoil to wind in 1988 alone. In the drought years of 1988-89, soil loss through wind and water was estimated at six billion tons per year.

The U.S. Department of Agriculture estimates that a six-inch loss of topsoil can reduce crop yields by 40 percent a year. Until topsoil is seen as a complex store of minerals and organic matter of great value, it will still be easy to abuse. Often soil has been seen only as a useful medium because it holds plants upright and can receive the water they need. The loss of essential dietary minerals has gone unnoticed. The remaining land has been forced to produce more food artificially and unsustainably. Salty, over-irrigated soils and creeping desert conditions are examples of the result—hardly conducive to good human nutrition.

KEEPING OUR SOIL MINERAL-RICH

In its natural state, quality soil is 45 percent minerals and is full of "good" bacteria. A teaspoon of good soil contains billions of living creatures. Soil is the major source of nutrients for most plants. Mineral-rich soil supports soil microbes that break down anything falling onto the soil, from dead leaves to picnic left-overs. In this way, matter is rotted down into its basic elements, including minerals, which then form part of the soil. This cycle keeps soil mineral-rich in a self-perpetuating cycle.

People often forget that bacteria are not usually disease agents, but actually perform very useful functions. Only when there are not enough bacteria to do the work required or the bacteria start to function where they are not needed does trouble begin. What prevents bacteria from devouring living plants? Plants are protected by a natural balance of fungi and bacteria. The fungi, called mycorrhiza, live along plant rootlets and secrete toxins which act against bacteria. The toxins, in a word, are antibiotics, just like the famous example produced from the *Penicillium* mold. By fending off bacteria, the mycorrhiza play an essential part in plant immunity and help create healthy crops.

When the uptake of minerals is out of balance, the result is deformity or deficiency. Mycorrhiza fungi help plants keep their mineral intake in balance. If mycorrhiza did not act as a buffer, plants would simply absorb minerals in proportion to the amounts found in soil. This would not necessarily match the plant's relative needs for each mineral. They perform this balancing action by binding needed minerals to protein, a process known as chelating. Chelation ensures that plants take in the minerals they need rather than the minerals in greatest quantity around them.

Healthy soil, then, is rich in bacteria that recycle matter into its basic elements which in turn help keep soil bacteria-rich. Plants benefit from the products of soil bacteria and don't get rotted down themselves because they are protected by fungi. Mycorrhiza fungi also protect plants from over- and underconsumption of the minerals they need. Such natural checks and balances in soil and plant life pay wonderful dividends to human beings in strong, healthy crops that can never be bettered by artificial, unnatural tinkering. And, of course, when we eat plants with the right balance of trace minerals, we're consuming the trace minerals essential for our own good health.

ARTIFICIAL FERTILIZERS AND PESTICIDES LEAD TO MINERAL LOSS

Topsoil loss is bad enough. The quality of the soil remaining is in many ways producing a slow starvation—not of calories, but of minerals. Since the industrial revolution and technological advances of the 19th and 20th centuries, farming itself has become an industry. Early scientific discoveries focused on boosting plant growth and killing agents of crop disease. Manmade fertilizers and pesticides did produce initial dramatic increases in crop yields and led to a large scale shift from traditional farming practices.

The invention of the tractor in the early 20th century distanced farmers even more from soil as the most vital resource of their work. Land began to be overworked and underfed at an unprecedented rate. It no longer seemed necessary to let fields lie fallow for a time or to dig crop remains back into the soil. Soil-rejuvenating crops known to host beneficial bacteria were no longer grown in years between crops reared for greater profit. Deficient soils unable to support livestock profitably were forced to grow crops for humans.

Soils in many areas have now become so deficient in enzymes, microbes, worms and insect life that crop remnants sit unrotted and do not become compost.

Science produced powerful chemicals in the form of

pesticides that could kill disease-producing organisms in plants. Pesticides changed the focus of farming from raising strong crops to treating sick ones or eliminating sources of sickness.

Chemical fertilizers are also part of the trend, substituting crop boosting for crop nurturing. Today, we pay the price of foods kept artificially free of disease and blemishes in mineral depletion and the risks that it brings.

Naturally caused inequalities will always exist in crops. Mineral variations are to be expected according to time of harvesting, climate and geology. However, the use of artificial fertilizers whose formulas are influenced by cost and profit rather than the actual needs of the soil in any given location has created unbalanced soil that is too high in some minerals and too low in others.

Chemical fertilizers contain relatively few minerals. This in itself leads to deficiencies in the "fertilized" plants. The chemical contents of artificial fertilizers are concentrated and acidic, typically mixtures of ammonia and nitrogen, and often strong enough to cause skin burns. Chemical fertilizers blaze a path through soil, destroying soil matter which would normally rot into a rich source of nutrients, and killing the microbes and other life that would achieve this. While chemical fertilizers cause the release of minerals from rocks in the soil, the microbes and mycorrhiza fungi disappear, making the released minerals unavailable to the plants. The same destructive process occurs with acid rain.

The combination of chemical fertilizer and pesticide use produces apparently healthy crops. The illusory appearance of large, good-looking fruits and vegetables masks the reality of severely compromised plant immunity brought about by inadequate nutrition. Nature would normally see to it that inferior plant life would not survive, but modern chemical treatments remove the fungi, insects and other life forms designed to carry out nature's work. Eventually, however, extreme natural conditions such as drought or frost reveal the serious inherent weaknesses of plants and soils treated with artificial fertilizers and we have farming disasters.

GOOD TRACE MINERALS DOWN, TOXIC ELEMENTS UP

Feed soil superphosphate fertilizer and crops grown on it will develop high levels of the toxic trace element cadmium. This has been known since work in the 1920s by soil scientist Dr. G. H. Earp-Thomas. Studies of trace elements show that under certain conditions toxic minerals can displace their beneficial cousins. Cadmium and essential zinc are good examples. This applies in the human body and soil alike. A plant growing in unbalanced soil containing high levels of cadmium will take up the toxic mineral in preference to zinc, actually blocking the plant's ability to absorb that essential element. The probable result for humans is an increase in uptake of cadmium, with its unfortunate ability to interfere with processes in the body that normally use zinc. The fact that Americans tend to be deficient in zinc owes much to this scenario.

The cadmium-zinc problem is only one of several examples. Where lead is present in high levels and calcium and magnesium are low, the body will take up lead instead of calcium and magnesium. This is a double whammy! The body is deprived of an essential mineral *and* poisoned with a toxic mineral.

Earp-Thomas also found that in the presence of too little sulfur a plant may take up toxic levels of selenium, and that chemical fertilizers high in phosphate will block the uptake of boron, a trace mineral increasingly accepted as essential. Studies have shown that boron decreases the loss of calcium and magnesium. Boron is also thought to be involved in the production of vitamin D and the synthesis of hormones, including estrogen.

It's important to remember that handy nutrition tables listing the amounts of vitamins and minerals in foods can only serve as rough guides. They cannot tell you, for example, if produce was grown in a mineral-balanced soil or a polluted soil. Nor can they give any indication of naturally occurring variations such as selenium deficiency in high-rainfall areas of the U.S. Chromium, iodine and selenium are three trace elements in particular that vary widely in soils from different geographic areas. What's more, many nutrition tables have not been updated in twenty years or more! In almost a century of practices which have continued to rob the soil of vital mineral content, even one year can make a difference to food values.

Studies show that natural farming produces foods of greater nutritional value than those grown with artificial fertilizers. Organic foods are also far less contaminated by chemicals. A study from the Universities of Maine and Vermont, published in 1987 in the *Journal of Food Quality*, found much lower levels of calcium, magnesium, beta-carotene and vitamin C in produce grown using chemicals than in naturally grown vegetables. Several studies have shown that the protein content of grains is increased when natural farming methods that maintain the mineral content of soil are used. Minerals play a key role in the formation of proteins. Molybdenum, for instance, is believed to be required by bacteria which convert nitrogen into a usable plant form. The resulting nitrates are used by plants as the basis of proteins.

CHAPTER 4

Food and Water as Mineral Sources

Your best source of minerals is the food you eat every day. Taking supplements is important too. It's a form of health insurance which acknowledges that nobody's diet is perfect, and that a certain percentage of the food we eat will not be supplying us with the vitamins and minerals our bodies need for optimal health.

COOKING FOR MINERALS

How you cook your food can make all the difference between getting the minerals you need and becoming deficient in minerals. You could buy a fresh, crisp head of organic broccoli, wash and chop it carefully, together with tender, organic carrots and new potatoes then drop them lovingly into a pan full of boiling water for ten minutes. You could do all this and watch the trace elements and other nutrients go up in steam and down the pan. Alternatively, you could steam your veggies for just enough time to create succulent rather than soggy servings and preserve the nutrients. Stir-frying can seal in nutrients when done fast, hot, started with water and finished off with a small amount of olive oil. If you use frozen vegetables, steam them without thawing. Of course, frozen meat and fish should always be thawed thoroughly before cooking.

For meat and vegetable cooking, stewing can be healthful as long as meats are browned first and drained of fat. Mineral and vitamin contents do leach out into broth, but will be consumed along with the finished stew.

Baking and roasting are both methods which cook using hot air. Bake or roast and you lose the fatty disadvantages of frying and the watery nutrient losses of boiling and steaming. Deep-frying only adds calories and potentially harmful chemicals. Cooking over charcoal and broiling bring the danger of contamination with chemicals in smoke from ignited fats. Broiling from above can help prevent this problem.

Microwave ovens should be reserved for rapid heating and defrosting. Long cooking with microwaves can change the chemistry of foods containing protein. Always use ceramic or glass containers for microwave preparation, as the heat causes chemicals to leach out from plastic and plastic wrap.

Foods lowest in fat content are foods richest in mineral nutrients. Selecting healthy foods and preparing them well prevents avoidable depletion of trace minerals, vitamins and other valuable nutrients.

WATER IS NOT THE MINERAL SOURCE IT USED TO BE

Running water is nature's primary delivery source of minerals. Its rushing, turbulent energy transports minerals from oceans and rocks to soil. It also leads to their existence in the highly available form of electrolytes. Research findings are now confirming that mineral absorption is highest when they are taken in dissolved form. Medical studies have shown this to be true of toxic minerals as well as dietary elements. One advantage that unpolluted, mineral-rich water has over foods is the absence of factors which can block mineral absorption. Such factors can be natural substances or chemical residues.

Ideally, drinking water should be an important source of trace elements. Unpolluted water from mountain and spring sources used to provide us with a range of beneficial minerals in a readily available form. Unfortunately, technology has created treated water for mass distribution that protects us from diseases such as cholera, but adds aluminum, chlorine and fluoride. Tap water is often also polluted with lead and copper from old plumbing. In high doses these substances compete with other important trace minerals for absorption.

In much of the industrialized world, municipal water treatment systems add aluminum to the water. Aluminum blocks other minerals in the body, it accumulates in the brain, liver, lungs and thyroid, and is a nerve poison in high amounts.

Chlorine, used to kill bacteria in water, is another toxic pollutant of tap water. In the gut, chlorine continues its sterilizing work, disturbing the balance of bacteria and potentially opening the door to an unfriendly overgrowth of organisms such as *Candida albicans.* Chlorine is also easily absorbed through the skin, especially in a hot shower when pores are open, adding to the body's overload.

Unless your water comes from a well that you check regularly for groundwater contaminants, I highly recommend that you purchase a water filter. A good one is expensive, but well worth the price for the health benefits, as you avoid chlorine, aluminum, benzene from petrochemical pollution, and many other potential hazards from treatment systems, industrial wastes and groundwater pollutants.

TRACE MINERALS AND THE FLUORIDATION CONTROVERSY

Many of what I call "health myths" have been sold to the American public in the name of profits. These myths creep in on the back of advertising, marketing, lobbying, political favors and kickbacks, and pretty soon they're taken as the gospel truth even though they're a pack of lies. There's the margarine-is-heart-healthy myth (the truth is that it has caused much more heart disease than it has prevented); there's the estrogen myth (it's more like the Grim Reaper than the Fountain of Youth), and there's the fluoride myth. I know, the common and seemingly irrefutable wisdom is that the number of cavities has been greatly decreased by the addition of fluoride to our drinking water and our toothpaste. I'm very sorry to say that it's not true, and that fluoride is most probably doing a great deal of harm.

Here's the story behind the story. During World War II we learned how to manufacture things from aluminum: airplanes, buildings and pots and pans, to name a few. We also greatly increased our production of chemical fertilizers. The down side of both these manufacturing processes was a byproduct called fluoride. Although fluoride is a trace mineral naturally occurring in our food, in anything but those trace amounts it's a more potent poison than arsenic. Disposing of the thousands of pounds of fluoride by-product became a major problem in American manufacturing. The manufacturers tried blowing it out their smokestacks, dumping it into rivers and burying it in the ground, but the immediate result was dead and deformed cows and other animals within miles of the smokestacks, rivers full of dead fish, and poisoned water aquifers. In fact its primary use was as a rat poison.

Finally, no doubt pushed by manufacturer's political pressure, the U.S. Public Health Service did a study claiming to show that one part per million of fluoride in water reduced tooth decay by 60 percent. Thus began the trickling of fluoride into our water supply.

The price of fluoride went up 1,000 percent almost overnight, and the problem of how to dispose of a potent toxin was solved. The practice of water fluoridation was further justified by more glowing studies claiming to show that communities using fluoridated drinking water had a much lower rate of tooth decay than those using unfluoridated water. The fluoride and cavity myth has been perpetuated by the fact that the rate of dental cavities has dropped steadily in the past thirty years, approximately the amount of time that our water has been fluoridated. So it must be good for us, right? Wrong.

The studies that were supposed to show how well fluoridated communities did are highly suspect. The original U.S. Public Health study on fluoridation was supposed to compare hundreds of communities, but the final study only included a few dozen, presumably those that fit the desired pro-fluoridation profile. And even those were flawed. For example, in the most widely cited study, two towns in Michigan were compared for dental cavities, but those children studied in the fluoridated community had higher incomes, received regular dental checkups, and agreed to brush their teeth twice a day. It wouldn't seem strange that they would have a lower rate of cavities, with or without fluoride!

"But," I hear you saying, "I had lots of cavities when I was a kid, and my kids hardly have any. It must be due to fluoride." Not so. In both fluoridated and unfluoridated areas in North America and Europe the decline in tooth decay has been the same for 30 years. This even holds true for entire countries in Europe that have not had fluoridated water or toothpaste. What has changed is that dental hygiene has improved, nutrition has improved, and access to dental care has improved. Studies do show a strong correlation between higher rates of tooth decay and lower economic status.

Japan and all of continental Europe either rejected the fluoride concept from the beginning or have stopped the practice. Most of Great Britain has also discontinued fluoridation, and Australia and New Zealand are in the process of reversing the trend. A 1994 study of virtually all New Zealand school children showed no benefit in dental health in fluoridated communities.

What's so bad about fluoride? There is good, solid evidence in eight reputable studies that fluoridated drinking water increases your risk of hip fractures by 20-40 percent. For a while it was thought that fluoride might actually help prevent osteoporosis. But long-term studies with hundreds of thousands of people proved the wisdom of checking things out thoroughly. There is a clear correlation between bone fractures and fluoridation. It turns out that while fluoride does create denser bone, it is poor-quality, structurally unsound bone that is actually more prone to fracture over time.

So much fluoride has been put into our water and toothpaste over the past 30 years that levels in our food chain are very high. Just by following a normal diet, the average person exceeds the recommended dose. Fluoride is a potent enzyme inhibitor that interferes with enzymes in the body, particularly in the lining of the intestines, causing stomach pain, gas and bloating. This enzyme-inhibiting effect also interferes with thyroid gland function. Some studies indicate that fluoride damages the immune system, leading to autoimmune disorders and arthritis. There is also evidence that communities with fluoridated water have a higher incidence of heart disease and higher rates of bone cancer in young men. Some 30 percent of children in fluoridated communities have fluorosis, a malformation of tooth enamel that causes discoloration (usually chalky white patches) and brittleness. This is a permanent change in the teeth that has also been associated with abnormal bone structure.

Advocates of putting fluoride in toothpaste and mouthwash argue that it is not swallowed, and therefore not ingested. However, fluoride is absorbed through the mucous membranes of the mouth, and young children do not have control over their swallowing reflex. There have been numerous reports of children poisoned by ingesting high levels of fluoride through school fluoride mouthwash programs, or fluoridated toothpastes full of sweeteners that kids want to swallow. (Please avoid both like the plague they are!) Who knows how many stomachaches in kids and adults alike have been caused by unknowingly ingesting too much fluoride?

While it is clear that fluoride can be helpful in the year or two when a child's adult teeth are growing in, there is absolutely no evidence that it is helpful before or after that time, and reams of evidence that it is harmful. A child's fluoride needs can be handled perfectly well by brushing with fluoride toothpaste for a few years. Other than that time of life, I recommend that you and your loved ones avoid fluoride in all forms, including toothpastes. This substance has crept into every link in our food chain, and the evidence is that even without fluoridated water and toothpaste we're getting a higher dose than is safe or recommended in our daily diets.

You can be thankful if you live in an unfluoridated community because it's not easy to get rid of fluoride in your tap water. Distillation and reverse osmosis are the only two reliable methods for removing fluoride. Other water filters may work at eliminating fluoride for a short period of time, but fluoride binds so strongly and quickly to filter materials such as charcoal, that the binding sites become fully occupied after a short time. If you are at a high risk for osteoporosis or heart disease, or if you have chronic digestive problems, I recommend you spend the money on a reverse osmosis water purification system.

REFINING FOODS EQUALS MINERAL ROBBERY

A better phrase than refined foods might be "nutrient-free." The obsession with convenience that has filled American lives since the '40s has brought increasingly dubious versions of food to TV trays across the land. When a food is refined, important parts of it are literally removed. White flour is produced by removing the outer husk of grains, consisting of the fibrous bran and germ, the part containing 95 percent of the nutrient value. The fiber is also removed from brown rice and whole sugar cane to give white variations of those foods. Advertising might lead us to believe that white sugar, rice and flour are "pure" foods. What they are is pure starch. "We need starch," you might say. This is true, but we also need essential minerals to aid in the digestion and processing of starch. The outer fiber of sugar and grains contains exactly the nutrients required to deal with the starch they surround.

Chromium found in the husk of grains is particularly needed in the processing of starch. Bran is itself fiber and contains other trace minerals like silicon and zinc as well as vitamin E and useful oils. Chromium is also found in unrefined sugar, where it is packaged with fiber and B complex vitamins. Fiber in products like unrefined flour and sugar provides bulk, acting as a check on excess consumption. Fiber also slows digestion and aids excretion of unwanted substances.

Pure starch taxes the body, as it stresses the pancreas and draws on stores of elements, especially chromium, needed for its digestion and absorption. What's more, as refined foods are processed, the body's acid/alkaline balance shifts toward acid. As the body works to restore its chemical balance it has to call even more on its mineral reserves. In this way, refining foods not only undersupplies but depletes trace minerals. Depletion is bad enough, but an additional result of eating only the inner core of rice and wheat grains is increased uptake of the element cadmium, which can accumulate to toxic levels. Cadmium is found largely in the central, starchy part of wheat and rice grains.

Unrefined wheat and rice are also packaged with zinc, mainly as part of their germ and bran. Zinc is absorbed by the body in preference to the toxic element, cadmium. Take away enough zinc and the cadmium is absorbed instead. White rice, white bread, white flour—all such refined products leave the door open to excess consumption of cadmium, which can inhibit the uptake of iron and block production of vitamin D.

Eating fresh, whole foods is like fitting the right keys into the locks of the body. Foods precooked, processed or refined in any other way may pick the locks of digestion and energy production, but they can damage them at the same time. Leave the convenience, fast and snack foods on the shelves and stick to whole, unrefined foods to keep your systems topped up with trace mineral levels and functioning smoothly.

"ENRICHED" FOODS ARE MINERAL POOR

U.S. law requires the addition of iron sulfate wherever iron and other minerals are removed during the processing of foods. Iron is an essential trace mineral with several valuable roles, particularly in the transportation of oxygen by the blood. I suppose the intention of this law is positive, but in practice it's almost useless, because iron sulfate is a form of iron that is not particularly well absorbed. In addition, absorption of the added iron in enriched food made with white flour or rice is likely to be blocked by other food additives or cadmium. Cadmium as an iron blocker is made available by the incidental removal of zinc during refining.

Does this make any sense to you? Iron is removed from foods, then replaced in questionable form, facing obstacles to its absorption. It is the same story or worse for other nutrients. More than thirty nutrients are removed from white, bleached flour. Four are added back, creating an "enriched" product. Ironically, the extracted nutrients are sold as animal feeds! To add insult to injury, manufacturers charge more for refined products sprayed with added nutrients. The only difference between one refined cereal and another can be sprayed-on vitamins and a higher price.

"Enriching" foods is nutritional nonsense. It plays havoc with the natural balances of trace elements established in foodstuffs. As seen with soil, mineral imbalances are perpetuated and worsened as nutrients are absorbed. The body has to scramble to provide minerals needed simply to digest foods robbed of their natural content, and it is not replenished. The selective replacement of a few nutrients ignores the fact that many work best when packaged with others that have not been restored.

Tinkering with the content of foods might pay the manufacturers, but it does not pay consumers in nutritional terms. Stay naturally enriched with trace minerals and other essential nutrients by steering clear of technologically "improved" food.

FIBER IS GOOD, BUT TOO MUCH IS NOT GOOD

Fiber is a perfect example of why moderation will keep you healthy in almost every aspect of your life. Fiber has been shown to be extremely important in the prevention of degenerative diseases including colitis, diverticulosis, ulcers and some cancers. Important minerals are packaged in the fiber around the energy-supplying starch in foods like rice and wheat. The body is adapted to absorb nutrients parceled in this way when they are consumed as part of a balanced diet.

The vast majority of Americans eat too many refined foods and don't get enough fiber. But too much isn't healthy either. Take in too much, and it will strip out trace elements and other nutrients. Fiber is largely indigestible and passes quickly out of the gut. Its ability to bind with toxins and other waste products is beneficial, in moderation. This ability simply extends too far when fiber levels are too high. It is highly unlikely that anyone will get too much fiber from the food they eat; most often the culprit is a fiber laxative or stimulant such as Metamucil (which is just psyllium with added colorings and sweeteners—the real thing is much, much cheaper and healthier).

If you're taking a fiber supplement such as psyllium, I recommend you take it first thing in the morning, at least half an hour before breakfast. This way it can stimulate and clean your digestive tract without taking nutrients with it. For the same reason, it's smart to take supplements at least an hour or two after taking a fiber supplement.

CHAPTER 5

Medicines and Mineral Depletion

I'll bet that when you take an antacid or an antibiotic, it never occurs to you that you could be creating a mineral deficiency or imbalance, but many, many over-the-counter (OTC) and prescription drugs interfere with mineral balance.

Some medications reduce mineral absorption, others cause minerals to be excreted in the urine in higher than normal quantities. Total intake of nutrients can change, too, as some drugs cause changes in appetite. In addition, the way a nutrient is used in the body can be altered by medications.

It is ironic that by disrupting nutrient uptake medications meant to heal the body can weaken it. One of the systems most impacted is the immune system, which requires vitamins and minerals for full protection against illness. A lack of nutrients may well lie behind a gap in the body's defenses which allows infection to take hold in the first place. Poor diet puts patients, particularly children and the elderly, at great risk from nutritional interference by drugs, especially if usage is long-term.

Research on drug and trace mineral interactions is sparse, but remember—wherever major minerals such as calcium, potassium and magnesium are lost, it's very likely that trace minerals are also being depleted.

Antacids are not a good source of calcium even though they may contain a great deal of it. In spite of advertising meant to convince you that stomach acid is your enemy, the truth is that heartburn and indigestion are most often caused by a *lack* of hydrochloric acid (HCl). Insufficient HCl leads to stomach churning and the fermentation of undigested food, which cause the food to be "urped" back up, burning the esophagus as it goes.

Taking antacids weakens or neutralizes acids for about an hour, relieving the symptoms, but often causing rebound heartburn or indigestion as the stomach tries to make up for the stomach acid it doesn't have by working overtime. In fact, in the long run, antacids will make heartburn and indigestion worse.

Antacids are advertised as being a good source of calcium, but this is misleading. The aluminum and magnesium in most antacids tend to bind with phosphate, which can result in calcium *depletion*! Weakened stomach acids cannot soften minerals, including calcium, arriving in the stomach. Minerals taken in are unlikely to be absorbed, and will almost certainly be excreted. The fact is that antacids can actually block calcium absorption and also tend to block iron absorption.

Some antacids deliver large amounts of compounds of aluminum, a trace element which can block mineral absorption and in large amounts can cause harm to the nervous system. Avoid taking antacids with citrus foods or drinks, as these increase the amount of aluminum absorbed. Aluminum hydroxides are the worst antacid culprits for blocking mineral absorption.

Used in too great amounts or for too long, antacids can produce vitamin and mineral deficiencies. If they do become necessary for extreme conditions, such as a true excess of HCl, their nutrient-blocking effects are lessened by taking them between meals or at night.

Most often I recommend that people with chronic heartburn and indigestion try taking betaine hydrochloride tablets before meals to aid digestion. Even simpler, just a warm glass of water with a tablespoon of apple cider vinegar can stimulate digestive juices and provide an acidic environment.

As an aside, please don't turn to the H2 blockers such as Tagamet, Pepcid and Zantac for heartburn and indigestion. They have a long list of side effects, and block the absorption of vitamin B12, which can cause symptoms of senility. Making these powerful drugs available over the counter is one of the most irresponsible actions the FDA has ever taken.

Antibiotics can be a powerful weapon against infection, but unfortunately they cannot distinguish between friend or foe. Antibiotics wipe out beneficial bacteria along with those causing harm. Take antibiotics and you will, for example, also destroy bacteria in the gut which produce the B-complex vitamin biotin. Mineral disruption can occur with the antibiotic Neomycin, which interferes with the absorption of calcium, iron, and potassium, as well as vitamin B12.

Some antibiotics interfere with the absorption of minerals, and the minerals interfere with the absorption of the antibiotic as well. Tetracycline blocks the absorption of dietary minerals by interacting with calcium, iron, magnesium and zinc, and taking these supplements will also block the action of the antibiotic.

Antibiotics known as quinolones will block the absorption of calcium, iron and zinc, and these minerals can also block the action of the antibiotic. Mineral supplements should be taken at least two hours away from tetracycline and the quinolones. Do not take antacids at the same time as these antibiotics either, because the calcium and magnesium may block their action.

As a general rule, problems with nutrient absorption end when the course of antibiotics ends. It is not advisable to take antibiotics for longer than about two weeks.

Anticonvulsants such as carbamazepine, phenobarbital, phenytoin and primidone block adequate production of vitamin D in the body. A lack of vitamin D leads the body to draw on calcium from bones instead of from dietary uptake. This is why long-term use of anticonvulsants can result in bone disorders. Another possible contributory factor in bone deformities caused by anticonvulsants is a lowering of blood and tissue levels of the trace mineral copper. Levels of zinc are also seen to drop over the long term when these drugs are used, compromising, among other functions, tissue formation and the immune system.

Antidepressants such as Fluoxetine, amoxapine, doxepin, imipramine and lithium carbonate may dampen the appetite and therefore indirectly cause nutrient deficiencies. Side effects such as abdominal cramps, diarrhea, dry mouth, nausea, and vomiting can occur with these types of drugs and with anti-anxiety medications like Librium and Valium. These symptoms can impair the absorption of nutrients. Long-term use of diazepam, for example, can disturb the balance of magnesium and calcium and increase the risk of bone disorders such as osteoporosis. Lithium disrupts copper absorption and may lead to a deficiency with long-term use.

Arthritis medications such as D-penicillamine can cause serious nutrient deficiencies, including mineral loss. Some of its side effects include an altered sense of taste, diarrhea, intestinal and digestive fluid problems, nausea, sores of the mouth and tongue, and vomiting, all of which can cause a loss of minerals. D-penicillamine reduces absorption of the trace element zinc, producing signs of clinical deficiency such as hair loss and skin changes. The drug binds to zinc and iron as well as other dietary minerals.

Aspirin can cause small amounts of blood to be lost in the stomach, and taking it regularly over a long period of time could result in enough blood loss to cause iron deficiency. I don't recommend that you take iron supplements, I recommend you avoid taking aspirin long-term! The pain killer indomethacin has the same problem.

Cholesterol-lowering drugs such as cholestyramine and colestipol lower the body's stores of iron as well as fat-soluble vitamins such as vitamins A, E and K, which are all protective against heart disease.

Corticosteroids such as cortisone and Prednisone are used to treat many illnesses, including arthritis and autoimmune diseases. They are also prescribed for skin problems, blood and eye disorders and asthma. Researchers conducted a study of 24 asthmatics using cortisone-type drugs and found the zinc levels were 42 percent lower than in patients not treated with corticosteroids.

Diuretics, frequently used in the treatment of high blood pressure and heart failure, can cause minerals to be lost in urine. Their effect is strongest with the beneficial minerals calcium, potassium and magnesium, but they also deplete the trace minerals iodine and zinc. Long-term diuretic use is definitely not encouraged. High blood pressure should always be vigorously treated first with lifestyle changes such as weight loss, exercise and a diet of nutrient-rich whole foods.

Laxatives turn nutrients into whistle-stop tourists of the intestine. Before they've had even a chance to inspect stomach or intestinal tract linings, nutrients are whisked away by laxatives. Even when nutrients do get to pause, laxatives like senna, and bisocodyl (Dulcolax) and phenolphthalein can interfere with the intestinal lining, possibly reducing nutrient uptake.

Mineral oil used as a laxative prevents absorption of vitamins A and D. Any laxative taken to excess can flush out large amounts of potassium, which can cause heart problems and muscle weakness.

Oral contraceptives tend to increase the levels of some vitamins and minerals, including copper, which in excess can cause a decrease in blood levels of iron and zinc. Studies have shown this type of medication can also lead to an increase in iron levels, possibly due to decreased menstrual flow.

Alcohol and tobacco. Alcohol is one our worst vitamin and mineral robbers. It depletes iron, selenium, zinc and magnesium, in addition to many other important nutrients. It also reduces the intake of minerals and nutrients in general by causing loss of appetite. Alcohol reduces absorption by damaging the lining of the small intestine and causes urinary loss of minerals. Alcoholic drinks like wine and whiskey are also relatively high in the toxic element cadmium, which is taken up in greater quantities when zinc levels are low.

While a glass of wine with dinner may be beneficial, tobacco is not suitable in any quantity! And remember that the harmful nutritional effects of tobacco extend to people breathing second-hand smoke. This is true especially because nonsmokers breathe in the unfiltered smoke which contains more poisons than the smoke breathed through a filtered cigarette. The trace element zinc and many other nutrients drop to low levels in smokers, impairing the immune system as well as the ability to detoxify the poisons being absorbed. Low zinc levels lead to a greater uptake and absorption of the trace element cadmium, which happens to be one of the toxins in tobacco smoke. Pregnant women who smoke are more likely to give birth to zinc-deficient babies.

CHAPTER 6

Keeping the Trace Minerals in Balance

Wouldn't life be a lot simpler if nutrition were only a matter of opening our mouths and pouring down a liquid super-food? Well, yes, but *we'd* be simpler, too, possibly drifting as a single cell in the ocean. As complex organisms, we have complex nutritional needs which are automatically supplied by foods in their natural forms. For example, whole-wheat bread brings the elements needed to digest it, and fruit delivers fast energy supported by the nutrients required to process it. Yet the production of our foods has to be literally rooted in properly balanced soils to ensure that nutrients blend as nature intended and health requires. Trace mineral interactions are examples of the way partnerships of nutrients abound. Research is increasingly showing the importance of nutrients in combination, which is powerfully demonstrated by the effects of trace minerals in and out of balance.

THE BODY WORKS TO CREATE OPTIMUM TRACE MINERAL LEVELS

The body is actually designed to maintain healthy levels of many trace minerals and hundreds of other biologically active chemicals. It performs constant, subtle adjustments in a wonderful, automatic effort to maintain balance, also known as homeostasis. (I think this word is misleading, because *stasis* means standing or stopping, and maintaining balance in the body is one of the most active processes I can think of.)

Excess trace elements are removed by preventing their absorption or triggering their excretion. Excretion occurs through feces, urine and sweat. Hair can also be a minor route of excretion for metallic trace minerals. Essential trace elements are nontoxic except in large amounts, and the body can temporarily tolerate a wide range between the highest and lowest levels associated with health. At low levels, the body can survive with an amount of a trace element sufficient for growth and maintenance, but insufficient for optimum function.

Mineral balance can be interfered with and overwhelmed, leading to inadequate or excess absorption. Normally the maintenance of optimum levels of trace minerals is affected by dietary consumption.

The intestines can reject excess amounts of trace minerals just as the kidneys can excrete them. However, both organs can only handle so much of any trace mineral. If that amount is exceeded, the body accumulates the mineral to poisonous levels.

TOXIC ELEMENTS CAN TAKE THE PLACE OF TRACE MINERALS

All elements, even oxygen, can become toxic at high enough levels. Extremely poisonous chemicals, such as mercury, are simply those that have toxic effects in very small amounts. Fortunately for the human race, nature has locked away many of the substances which are harmful in low amounts. Humans, however, have been uncovering them at increasing rates, mining uranium and other heavy metals and minerals. We are also exposed to unprecedented levels of lead through car exhaust, and cadmium through poor agricultural processes. This has increased the need for trace elements required to help protect the body and process noxious chemicals. It has also led to a greater chance that toxic chemicals may be absorbed instead of essential trace elements.

Essential trace minerals belong to different families of elements which include toxic cousins. Just as with plants, if not enough of a particular trace element is present, the body will take up its nearest available cousin. Illness can be caused, for example, when cadmium displaces zinc, changing or inactivating enzymes. Disease conditions can occur when insufficient iodine causes the thyroid gland to take up sodium fluoride instead. Iodine pills were issued by the Polish government after the nuclear disaster of Chernobyl in 1986. This was to try to prevent an uptake of radioactive iodine in place of essential iodine.

The best prevention of toxic element uptake is to avoid exposure by buying organic foods and living in an unpolluted environment. A healthy diet also protects you from harmful elements by maintaining trace element levels, filling any gaps a toxic cousin might fit. Optimum levels of trace elements also aid the body's detoxifying mechanisms.

HOW ESSENTIAL TRACE ELEMENTS INTERACT

The interaction of several trace minerals and other nutrients requires a cautious and intelligent approach to supplementation. The human body is geared to receive nature's own balanced recipes of nutrients that exist in individual foods. Ideally, trace elements and other nutrients should be readily available from whole food sources without major concerns about their correct proportions or partners. Sadly, a compromised and polluted environment leads to an unbalanced uptake of nutrients and unnatural toxins. This generates a need for wisely chosen supplements and diet. Awareness of the types of stress which use up trace minerals helps to promote use of supplements at the right time. Supplies of zinc, for example, are run down with infection, and iron will be lost with extensive bleeding.

A good general rule is to avoid taking higher-than-recommended doses of any one mineral without taking into account the effect it will have on other minerals, especially when taking them long-term. Trace mineral interactions include the following:

Cobalt and molybdenum. Molybdenum antagonizes cobalt.

Cobalt and iodine. Cobalt antagonizes iodine.

Copper and molybdenum. Molybdenum may alter copper absorption, but copper is also believed to work against molybdenum.

Copper and selenium. Copper is believed by some investigators to be a selenium antagonist, probably competing for absorption.

Iron and magnesium carbonate. Excessive magnesium carbonate could reduce the absorption of iron. (Note: Magnesium carbonate is not a good magnesium supplement since it is not easily absorbed.)

Iron, copper, manganese and zinc. Take too much of one and you may cause a deficiency in another of these trace minerals, creating an increased risk of infection and other diseases. These elements compete for absorption in the small intestine. When in balance, copper enhances the absorption and utilization of iron. Zinc in particular competes against copper for absorption.

CHAPTER 7

Food Sources of Essential Trace Minerals

The food values found in tables do not account for variations caused by climate, geology and time of harvesting, or those caused by chemical farming. However, they do provide basic information about which foods are usually comparatively high in certain trace minerals and other nutrients. It's a good idea to hedge against depletion of nutrients in any one food by eating a range that in theory supplies the content you are looking for.

Boron. Good sources are fruits and vegetables.

Chromium. Good sources are black pepper, thyme, cheese, lean meat, and whole grain cereals.

Cobalt. Good sources are meats and other foods of animal origin.

Copper. Good sources are shellfish, especially oysters, avocado, fish, poultry, dark green leafy vegetables, cooked soybeans, dried peas and other legumes, nuts, bananas and other fruits, whole-grain bread and cereals and cooked carrots.

Iodine. Good sources include iodized salt, seafood and seaweed.

Iron. Good sources (all better than spinach) include red meats, brewer's yeast, kelp, lima beans, chickpeas, duck, shellfish, molasses, wheat bran, parsley and apricots.

Manganese. Good sources are whole grains, nuts, shellfish and milk. Given soil that is not too alkaline, fruit and green vegetables can be moderate sources of manganese.

Molybdenum. Good sources are whole grains, dark green leafy vegetables, peas, beans, and milk. Crops grown on depleted soil can have molybdenum levels up to 500 times lower than plants grown on soil rich in this mineral.

Selenium. Good sources are brewer's yeast, broccoli, cabbage, celery, cucumbers, fish, garlic, whole grains, mushrooms, and poultry. However, selenium levels vary greatly in soils. As a general rule, soils in the Western states are lower in selenium than soils in Eastern ones.

Zinc. Good sources are fish, meat, oysters, and whole grains.

KELP

Kelp, a seaweed, is an excellent source of minerals. It contains 23 minerals, the most important of which are present in the percentages shown:

Iodine	0.15-0.20%	Magnesium	0.76%
Calcium	1.20	Sulfur	0.93
Phosphorus	0.30	Copper	0.0008
Iron	0.10	Zinc	0.0003
Sodium	3.14	Manganese	0.0008
Potassium	0.63		

Vitamins present in kelp are: vitamin B2, niacin, choline and carotene. Algenic acid is also present. This remarkable food contains more vitamins and minerals than any other substance. All these nutrients have been assimilated by the growing plant.

Kelp, because of its natural iodine content, acts to normalize the thyroid gland. Therefore, thin people with thyroid trouble may gain weight by using kelp, and obese people with thyroid trouble may lose weight.

If you need a good supply of highly absorbable minerals, try taking kelp supplements.

CHAPTER 8

The *Good* Trace Minerals from A to Zinc

Minerals work in partnership with hormones, enzymes, amino acids and vitamins. They are required to build and maintain the structure of the body. They are involved in the breakdown of food during digestion, and some are instrumental in maintaining fluid balance inside cells. Those that are currently considered essential for human nutrition are calcium, phosphorus, iron, potassium, selenium, and magnesium. In reality, however, many more minerals are needed to maintain optimal health. Chromium, cobalt, copper, zinc and manganese are important in their own right, even though we only require them in very small amounts.

Unless you are trying to correct a specific nutritional deficiency under the supervision of a health care professional, minerals should only be taken in the recommended doses, as an excess can cause just as many problems as a deficiency.

Let's take a closer look at the trace minerals you should be getting in your daily vitamin program.

BORON

Boron is a trace mineral that helps retard bone loss and works with calcium, magnesium and vitamin D to help prevent osteoporosis (brittle bones). Some studies suggest that a boron deficiency may aggravate arthritis and other degenerative joint conditions. Boric acids and borates have been used medicinally for centuries as disinfectants and to treat burns.

As I mentioned earlier in the book, we tend to be deficient in boron, because the use of superphosphate fertilizers blocks its uptake by plants.

According to boron researcher Forrest H. Nielsen of the Department of Agriculture's Grand Forks Human Nutrition Research Center, calcium cannot be properly metabolized without boron. He fed a low-boron diet (less than 0.32 milligram per day) to five men, five postmenopausal women on bone-preserving estrogen therapy, and four postmenopausal women not on estrogen, for 63 days. Then, for the next 49 days, they continued on the low-boron diet, but added a daily 3-mg supplement of boron.

On the low-boron diet, blood levels of calcium decreased, along with other nutrients that affect bone health. When boron was added back in, all these measures improved, and copper levels improved as well.

You can take 1-3 milligrams of boron daily—not more than that—if you are at risk for osteoporosis. Otherwise, you can get boron in a healthy diet. Boron is abundant in pears, apples and grapes, and is also found in nuts, green, leafy vegetables and legumes such as soy beans.

CHROMIUM

Chromium is one of our most important trace minerals, and one of the most depleted. It works with insulin in the metabolism of sugar and helps the body utilize protein and fats. Taken in conjunction with exercise, chromium helps the body burn off fat more efficiently. It is best to take chromium in the form of chromium picolinate. Chromium also helps prevent and lower high blood pressure.

Recent studies suggest that chromium may help athletes by regulating the body's use of glycogen during exercise. In one study, weight lifters using chromium supplements had greater muscle and weight gains than a group given a placebo. In another study, chromium supplements lowered blood cholesterol levels.

It is also very important to those with blood sugar and insulin imbalances, such as diabetics. Chromium is necessary for glucose to enter the cells, so it is essential in the efficient burning of carbohydrates. In fact, a chromium deficiency may cause adult-onset diabetes, especially in older people.

I know the people who make those awful bottled "natural" fruit drinks and teas aren't going to like me for saying this, but I suspect that the steep rise in our consumption of high-fructose corn syrup has contributed to the rise in diabetes by depleting chromium. (As our consumption of high-fructose corn syrup has risen 250 percent in the past 15 years, our rate of diabetes has increased approximately 45 percent in about the same time period.) According to studies done at the Agriculture Department's Human Nutrition Resource Center, fructose consumption causes a drop in chromium, as well as raising "bad" LDL cholesterol and triglycerides, and impairing immune system function.

According to researchers, giving people with elevated blood sugar a chromium supplement will result in a significant drop in blood sugar in 80 to 90 percent of those people.

Chromium may also be important for skin health. In a study reported in *Medical Hypotheses,* when nine patients with acne were given two teaspoons daily of high-chromium yeast containing 400 micrograms of chromium, their acne rapidly cleared up.

Please don't be scared away from chromium by recent media reports about it. Taking chromium picolinate supplements of 100 to 600 mcg daily is not the same as exposing hamster cells in a test tube to 5,000 to 6,000 times that dose every day, nor is it the same as factory workers breathing chromium dust.

Most Americans are actually deficient in chromium, and at the recommended doses it is very safe and very effective in helping stabilize blood sugar as well as helping burn fat during exercise and producing lean muscle tissue.

You can take 200 mcg of chromium daily, depending on your needs. Food sources of chromium include brewer's yeast, whole grains, nuts, molasses and cheese.

COBALT

Cobalt is a component of vitamin B12, and as such is a stimulant to the production of red blood cells, and is necessary for normal cell growth and healthy nerve tissue. A deficiency of cobalt/B12 can cause anemia. Although a deficiency of cobalt is rare, it can occur in vegetarians, since cobalt is mainly found in meat and shellfish in the form of vitamin B12. Cobalt can also replace other trace minerals in enzyme reactions, and is part of the enzyme action involved in forming some antioxidants.

COPPER

Copper and zinc balance each other in the body, and a deficiency of one can cause an excess of the other. Copper is necessary for absorption and utilization of iron and the formation of red blood cells.

Copper works as a catalyst in the formation of red blood cells and is present in the hemoglobin molecule. It also plays a role in maintaining the skeletal system. Copper is essential before iron can be utilized and is necessary to prevent anemia. It is an important partner to vitamin C in the synthesis of collagen. You don't usually need to add copper to your diet. An excess can cause hair loss, insomnia, irregular menses and depression.

FLUORIDE

Fluoride helps protect teeth from decay and may help protect against osteoporosis. Too much causes discolored teeth and continued overuse of it may lead to bone fractures, abnormal bony growths, heart disease and digestive disorders. Most Americans get excessive fluoride in their normal diet, just by drinking tap water, sodas, and other commercial products made with fluoridated water. I don't recommend that you supplement fluoride in your diet. See page 21 for more about the fluoridation controversy.

IODINE

As far back as Hippocrates, physicians have known that something in seaweed and seafood prevents goiter, an enlargement of the thyroid gland. Iodine is the key component in a thyroid hormone called thyroxin, and a lack of it causes the thyroid gland to enlarge. Since the thyroid regulates our metabolism—how fast we use energy—it is an essential trace mineral. And yet, it is a trace mineral found in the sea, and rarely inland. Many inland areas of the world are still deficient in iodine and suffer from diseases relating to improper thyroid function.

Iodine is necessary for proper growth, and promotes healthy hair, nails, skin and teeth. A deficiency of iodine in pregnant women can cause retardation in their children, and children deficient in it may become retarded. A deficiency of vitamin A can make iodine deficiency even worse.

Iodine deficiency can be caused by eating too many vegetables in the cabbage family (kale, cauliflower, turnips) without a sufficient intake of iodine. A substance in these vegetables blocks the uptake of iodine. Disease conditions can occur when insufficient iodine causes the thyroid gland to take up sodium fluoride instead.

Sufficient iodine levels also confers some protection against radiation damage, as a lack of it will cause the thyroid to take up the radioactive trace elements instead. As mentioned earlier, it was for this reason that the Polish government distributed iodine pills after the Chernobyl nuclear disaster.

An oversupply of iodine can cause or aggravate acne in adolescents. Some researchers speculate that this is caused when the excess iodine is excreted through the pores, irritating the skin.

Seafoods are very high in iodine, and it is added to most table salt. Kelp is a good source of natural iodine. You should be getting 150 mcg or 0.15 mg of iodine daily as part of your food or in your multivitamin. Pregnant and nursing women should be getting 175-200 mcg daily.

IRON

Iron is required in the manufacture of hemoglobin, a component of blood, and helps carry oxygen in the blood. It works with many enzymes in biochemical reactions in the body, and to be used efficiently must also have copper, cobalt, manganese and vitamin C. B-complex vitamins such as B1, B6, biotin, folic acid and B12, all work with iron to produce rich red blood.

Women need more iron than men because of the

loss of blood during the menstrual cycle, and their need for iron is increased during pregnancy and breast feeding.

In excess, iron is not efficiently excreted from the body. It can accumulate in tissue and become toxic. Recent research has shown that excessive amounts of iron in the tissues raises the risk of heart disease. Some researchers theorize that part of the reason a woman's risk of heart disease increases after menopause is that she is not losing iron every month during menstruation. Although iron is an essential mineral, it is important not to take too much iron in supplement form. A deficiency can cause a specific disease called iron deficiency anemia.

The most noticeable warning sign of anemia, a sign of iron deficiency, is fatigue. If you are getting plenty of rest, but still feel tired and lacking in energy, your body could be telling you that you are becoming anemic. The hair, skin and nails also show the effects of anemia. The skin tends to wrinkle more. Fingernails and toenails become brittle and break easily, and become tender. Hair becomes dry and lacks luster. Skin color becomes paler, even pasty and gray. The mouth and tongue begin to feel sore and tender.

Since the most available sources of absorbable iron are meat, vegetarians are at a greater risk of becoming iron-deficient.

Sufficient iron levels are essential for top athletic performance. Since iron plays a role in delivering oxygen to the muscles, iron-poor blood can cause less efficient use of muscles and fatigue. Studies have shown that women athletes in particular may benefit from iron supplements, even when iron levels test as normal. A study of high-school cross-country runners found 45 percent of the female runners and 17 percent of the male runners had low iron levels during the competitive season. Another study of 100 female college students showed that 31 percent had iron deficiency. The population most susceptible to iron deficiency is young women who are dieting to keep their weight down, and also exercising strenuously. For young athletes, keeping the body well stocked with iron can improve endurance and keep red blood cells optimally healthy.

Iron supplements can cause constipation, diarrhea, nausea and poor absorption of zinc. Your best bet is to eat plenty of iron-rich foods and keep iron supplements low. In fact, I don't recommend iron supplements except for young women and possibly pregnant women as needed, unless blood tests show low iron levels. Most iron deficiency anemia can be cured by proper diet. If you need iron supplementation, 10 mg daily is a reasonable amount to take. If you want to take more, please do so under the guidance of a health care professional who can measure your iron levels.

LITHIUM

Lithium is a trace mineral only recently studied, and is not needed in significant enough amounts in the body to be supplemented. However, lithium has been used successfully for years to treat manic depression, now known as bipolar mood disorder. It is a treatment that must be used with care, because it interacts with other substances, and can cause kidney damage and death if it accumulates to a toxic level.

Some researchers have used lithium to successfully treat those attempting to withdraw from alcohol, cocaine and other drugs.

The two most common side effects of lithium are weight gain and fatigue, which may be caused by reduced thyroid function, even though thyroid tests are normal. Lithium may also cause a deficiency of folic acid, which can increase the risk of heart disease and some cancers, and cause a deficiency of vitamin B12. A report from the National Institutes of Health suggests that taking the B vitamin inositol with lithium may reduce the side effects.

Lithium also replaces sodium when there is a sodium deficiency, which can upset the delicate balance of fluid in the cells, causing edema, nausea and vomiting.

Many arthritis and pain medications interfere with lithium excretion and can cause a toxic buildup. These include aspirin, ibuprofen (Advil, Motrin), naproxen (Aleve), and indomethacin (Indocin). Both the thiazide diuretics (furosemide, bumetanide) and the potassium-sparing diuretics (spironolactone, triamterene) used to treat high blood pressure can also raise lithium levels dangerously. The same is true of the heart drugs known as ACE inhibitors, such as captopril, enalapril and quinapril. The anticonvulsant carbamazepine (Tegretol) can make lithium more effective in some people, but in others can cause toxicity.

I recommend that you use lithium only under the guidance of a health-care professional. If you are taking it and experience nausea, diarrhea, muscle weakness, call your doctor immediately.

MANGANESE

Manganese is another trace mineral that we're learning more about every day. It is an important trace mineral that activates numerous enzymes, and is related to proper utilization of vitamins B1, E and iron. Manganese is also involved with thyroid function, the central nervous system, and digestion of proteins. It increases levels of the antioxidant SOD (superoxide dismutase).

Very little manganese is stored in the body, making it an important mineral to include in a supplement program. Too much manganese interferes with iron absorption, and conversely, too much iron can reduce manganese levels.

Although manganese deficiency is not well studied, some of the symptoms of manganese deficiency are middle ear problems, reduced fertility, retarded growth and low blood sugar.

A study of trace metals conducted during autopsies of 32 people, of whom 16 had blocked arteries, showed that those with the heart disease had low copper and manganese levels in the damaged arteries.

Manganese plays a role in the breakdown of collagen, and a deficiency can cause dermatitis; it can reduce levels of "good" HDL cholesterol, and cause bone loss and bone instability. A study of women with osteoporosis showed that they had low manganese levels, and rodent studies indicate that it is a crucial mineral in the formation of strong, normal bone.

Researchers all over the world have reported success in treating schizophrenia with manganese, and some theorize that it plays an important role in stabilizing nerve transmissions. It has also been used to treat seizures, and this may be connected to its important role in the middle ear.

Manganese is one of the important trace minerals removed when grains are refined. The prevalence of *nutrition-free* refined foods in America has made manganese deficiency common. Since manganese competes with calcium, it should be taken separately as a supplement.

I recommend that women at risk for osteoporosis add 5-10 mg of manganese to their daily supplements, and other adults include 2-5 mg daily.

MOLYBDENUM

This trace mineral was once considered toxic because miners inhaling it became ill. However, we now know that it is important to human health in very small quantities. It is used by blue-green algae and other plant life to turn nitrogen into a useable compound essential to all life, so its presence is foundational to life as we know it.

A deficiency of molybdenum has been linked to age-related cataracts and cancer of the stomach and esophagus. It is one of the trace elements necessary for the metabolism of iron, and it plays important roles in at least three enzyme systems having to do with the metabolism of fats, carbohydrates and proteins.

There is evidence that sufficient molybdenum is important to the formation of strong teeth, which makes sense since it is a component of tooth enamel, and it is vital to the normal development of the fetus.

Since molybdenum and copper compete with each other, an excess of one can cause a deficiency of the other. Excess sulfur can also cause a deficiency of molybdenum.

Molybdenum is one of the trace minerals stripped out of refined grains, and depleted from many soils. I recommend that you include 100-250 mcg of molybdenum in your daily vitamin intake.

SELENIUM

Selenium is a trace mineral found in very small amounts in the body. However, its role in maintaining our health is anything but small. I have been telling my readers about this mineral for 20 years. In 1957, Dr. Klaus Schwarz and Dr. C. M. Katz established that selenium is essential to life, even though it is needed in very small quantities, but it was not until 1990 that it was designated as a recommended dietary allowance (RDA) mineral. This means that your body must have this mineral daily. If we need selenium in such small amounts, why do we need to add it to our diets? White bread is one answer. Processing grain to produce white flour robs it of 75 percent of its selenium content.

Selenium could be called the "anticancer" mineral. Over and over again population studies have shown that people living in areas containing plenty of selenium in the soil have lower rates of cancer, and those living in areas with selenium-depleted soil have higher rates, especially of colon cancer.

Selenium is an antioxidant that also stimulates the immune system. A deficiency can lead to impaired immune function and reduced T-cell counts.

It works synergistically with vitamin E, each enhancing the actions of the other. Selenium is found in high concentrations in semen, and men seem to need more of this mineral than women. A selenium deficiency can cause dandruff, dry skin and fatigue, and may be associated with the development of cataracts.

Selenium is important in male hormone regulation and is found in large amounts in the prostate. Blood levels of both zinc and selenium are low in men who have prostate cancer. Men who live in areas where the soil is rich in selenium tend to have lower rates of prostate cancer.

Selenium is protective against heavy metal exposure, specifically to mercury, it is important in the formation of the antioxidant glutathione, and has been associated with reductions in heart disease.

Selenium also aids in keeping youthful elasticity to your tissues, can help alleviate hot flashes and other menopausal symptoms, and helps in the treatment and prevention of dandruff.

If you're over the age of 50 I suggest you supplement your diet with up to 200 mcg of selenium daily.

VANADIUM

Vanadium is a mineral mainly stored in our bones and fat. Although no human deficiency of vanadium has ever been identified, in test animals a deficiency caused impaired growth of teeth, bones and cartilage, thyroid changes, decreased overall growth, and fluid retention. This mineral can also be used to build up teeth, bones, cartilage and even muscle. It stimulates cell division, but also has anticarcinogenic properties.

A substance called vanadyl sulfate, which is derived from vanadium, is used to increase muscle growth and development, and appears to make muscles larger and denser more rapidly than would normally be the case.

Vanadyl sulfate is also very important in the treatment of diabetes. It helps insulin work more efficiently, and that may be why it also lowers cholesterol and triglyceride levels.

If you have diabetes, I don't recommend long-term high doses of vanadium, but you can use it to help stabilize your blood sugar, and then cut back. Try starting with 6 mg daily and work your way up to 100 mg daily until you get results. Once you begin having results, stay at that dose for up to three weeks and then taper back gradually to 6-10 mg daily.

Normally it is not necessary to include vanadium as a dietary supplement.

ZINC

Think of zinc as a traffic policeman, directing and overseeing the efficient flow of body processes, the maintenance of enzyme systems, and the integrity of our cells. It is a tiny but powerful catalyst which is absolutely essential for most body functions.

Zinc is a trace mineral found in the thyroid gland, hair, finger- and toenails, nervous system, liver, bones, pancreas, kidney, pituitary glands, blood and in the male reproductive fluid or semen. It is the prime element in male hormone production. Zinc is a constituent of insulin, which is necessary for the utilization of sugar. It also assists food absorption through the intestinal wall.

Zinc governs the contractility of our muscles, stabilizes blood, and maintains the relationship of acidity and alkalinity in the blood and other fluids. Zinc is essential for the synthesis of protein and in the action of many enzymes. A lack of zinc can cause increased fatigue, susceptibility to infection and injury and a slowdown in alertness and scholastic achievement.

Zinc exerts a normalizing effect upon the prostate and a lack of the mineral can produce testicular atrophy and prostate trouble. Zinc is necessary for the proper function of the prostate gland. In men, higher concentrations of this mineral are found in the prostate than anywhere else in the body. A recent study looked at zinc supplementation in young men, and found that when plasma zinc levels were low, there was a corresponding drop in testosterone. There have been many clinical studies showing that zinc supplementation can reduce the size of the prostate gland, along with troublesome symptoms.

Zinc supplements during pregnancy appear to promote an increase in birth weight. When you exercise vigorously, you lose a lot of zinc, so it's important for athletes to take a zinc supplement.

Most zinc available in foods is lost in processing. For example, 80 percent of the zinc in white bread is destroyed by processing. White spots or bands on the fingernails may indicate zinc deficiency.

Zinc supplements can be taken as lozenges, and in that form can cut down the length and severity of colds and flus, especially when combined with vitamin C.

Zinc is important in maintaining clear skin. Zinc stimulates antibody production to help fend off invading organisms on the skin surface. Some adolescent acne may be caused by a zinc deficiency.

As with all minerals, please don't take zinc in excess as it will cause other imbalances in your body. Zinc works best in combination with vitamin A, calcium and phosphorus.

I recommend that all men take up to 15-30 mg of zinc daily, and include zinc-rich foods in the diet such as oysters (well cooked please!), lamb chops and wheat germ. Pumpkin seeds are a good source of zinc.

Pregnant women and athletes can take 15-30 mg daily.

Everyone else should include 5-15 mg of zinc in their daily vitamin supplements.

CHAPTER 9

The *Bad* Trace Minerals and How to Avoid Them

The following trace minerals I have labeled as "bad" because, although they exist in the body in extremely small amounts, they can cause toxicity in minute doses, some as small as a few parts per million. Even the "good" trace minerals are only beneficial in very small amounts, and become toxic in large amounts. The toxic metals tend to accumulate in the body, increasing their potential for toxicity. Some can enter the brain, causing serious biochemical imbalances. Pollution by industrial wastes, car exhaust, farming with artificial fertilizers, pesticides and fungicides, copper and lead in pipes, polluted ground water, as well as cooking and eating utensils made of these substances, has created an environment where metal poisoning is common in the industrialized world.

It's easy to become frightened after reading about the pervasiveness of these metals in the environment and the extent of the damage they can do to the body, and there is certainly cause for concern and watchfulness. Your best ally is education; finding out what the sources of these metals are, and then avoiding them as best you can. A single exposure to toxic trace minerals is unlikely to cause serious illness unless it is a very large dose. Most poisoning occurs through small doses over time.

Exposure to toxic trace minerals can be insidious, because the symptoms may be generalized and not severe enough to warrant a visit to the doctor or proper blood testing by a doctor, yet be severe enough to cause chronic fatigue, headaches, dizziness and/or mental and emotional symptoms such as irritability, confusion, memory loss, hyperactivity and even violent behavior.

According to research reported by the American Society For Reproductive Medicine, air pollution with heavy metals may be an unsuspected cause of infertility. Exposure to cadmium, nickel, manganese and zinc at concentrations not high enough to be directly toxic can produce changes in sperm that cause infertility. Male infertility is increasing at an alarming rate. Some estimates put it at 1 percent per year. (Exposure to hormone-altering pesticides is also playing a role in male infertility.)

A balanced nutritious diet, drinking plenty of clean water, moderate exercise and a daily multiple vitamin will make a big difference in your body's ability to detox and clear out any overload of toxic minerals. Getting the "good" minerals in your daily vitamin regimen is particularly important because many of the toxic trace minerals replace good minerals such as calcium, iron and zinc.

ALUMINUM

Thanks to industrial pollution and the widespread use of aluminum in foods, medicines, municipal water treatment and cosmetics, people living in industrialized nations are exposed to much higher levels of this metal than is safe.

Although it is the third most abundant element in the earth's crust, aluminum is only found in very small amounts in plants and animals. Up to a point, our bodies are well equipped to safely excrete most of the aluminum we ingest. But in larger doses it becomes toxic, causing bone abnormalities, muscle weakness, loss of balance and coordination, memory loss and depression. Because aluminum interferes with the absorption of important minerals such as selenium, magnesium and calcium, its toxic effects can include the deficiency diseases caused by lack of these minerals.

The fact that aluminum's toxicity remains controversial has more to do with greed and politics than a lack of scientific research. Aluminum in excess is clearly a poison, but it is also the third most used metal product in the United States. This means that the aluminum lobbyists are well endowed and powerful enough to discourage government action that might decrease our exposure to aluminum.

Because aluminum is so pervasive in the environment, it pays to avoid it whenever possible, because even then you're likely to be getting regular overdoses of it.

Aluminum and Alzheimer's Disease

Although research into the connection between Alzheimer's disease and aluminum remains controversial, it is clear from half a dozen good population studies that those with higher levels of aluminum in their water supply have higher levels of Alzheimer's. Rats whose brains are injected with aluminum have symptoms similar to those of Alzheimer's. A Johns Hopkins University study found that those patients undergoing hemodialysis who had increased levels of aluminum also had decreased levels of cognitive brain function. The authors of that study theorized that aluminum may interfere with the brain's ability to use glucose, and thus its ability to produce important brain chemicals such as acetylcholine.

It may also be that some people have a genetic susceptibility to brain damage caused by a combination of factors, including aluminum. Whatever the cause or combination of causes, aluminum is clearly implicated in Alzheimer's disease, and for that reason alone I would recommend you avoid it.

Sources of Aluminum

One of the most pervasive sources of aluminum is simply industrial byproducts, blown out smokestacks, dumped into rivers and waste sites and trickling into our water aquifers. The secondary effect of industrial air pollution is acid rain, which contains high levels of aluminum which leaches through the soil into ground water over time.

Aluminum also enters water through municipal treatment plants because aluminum sulfate (alum) is used to clarify the water. To add insult to injury, there is some evidence that adding fluoride to the water makes the aluminum even more toxic by making it more difficult to excrete. Aluminum fluoride also crosses the blood-brain barrier more easily, exposing the brain to increased levels of both aluminum and fluoride. Ironically, the sodium fluoride pumped into America's water supplies is a waste product of aluminum manufacturing!

Aluminum is very commonly used in processed foods as an emulsifier, to prevent clumping, and to whiten ingredients. It is found in processed flours of all kinds, baking powder, processed fruits and vegetables, and table salt. There are literally dozens of variations on aluminum additives, but some of the more common ones you'll find on food labels are: alum, aluminum potassium sulfate, sodium aluminum phosphate, sodium silicon aluminate, aluminum calcium silicate, potassium alum, aluminum stearate and aluminum hydroxide. Suffice it to say that anything with the word aluminum in it counts.

Probably the next most common source of aluminum is antacids. Antacid users can easily consume 5 grams (5,000 mg) of aluminum per day. Since 150 mg a day is considered a safe level of aluminum consumption, antacids represent a major source of aluminum overdose. Indigestion and heartburn become more common as we age, and antacid use and abuse rises steeply in people over the age of 50. (See my book in this series, *Dr. Earl Mindell's What You Should Know About Fiber and Digestion,* for specifics on preventing and treating indigestion and heartburn naturally.) As we age, we accumulate heavy metals in our tissues, so throwing any additional burden on top of an already overloaded system may be pushing some senior citizens into symptoms of senility by blocking essential trace minerals such as selenium, and causing brain chemistry changes. Antacids also interfere with the absorption of nutrients, so I recommend that you avoid them except for occasional use, and then use antacids that don't contain aluminum.The most common type of aluminum in antacids is aluminum hydroxide, which is transformed by hydrochloric acid in the stomach to aluminum chloride, which is easily absorbed in the intestines. Drinking citrus juice such as orange or grapefruit, or taking vitamin C within an hour or two of taking an antacid can greatly increase the absorption of aluminum.

Aluminum is also put into deodorants designed to be absorbed through the skin, creating daily source of aluminum consumption. Toothpaste is another source of aluminum compounds that can be avoided. Your local health food store will have aluminum-free deodorants and toothpastes.

Although aluminum pots and pans are not as large a source of aluminum as food additives, they remain a daily source of aluminum consumption for those who use them. Acidic foods such as tomatoes and coffee leach more aluminum from pots and pans, and there is evidence that as they age they corrode, increasing levels of aluminum ingested. It's safer for your health in the long run to use stainless steel pots or pans with copper or aluminum outer bottoms to conduct heat evenly, or you can use glass cookware.

ARSENIC

When I think of arsenic I think of Victorian-era detectives on the trail of an arsenic poisoning, and indeed for centuries it was one of the most popular ways to kill someone else or commit suicide. Arsenic accumulates in the body, so taking very small amounts over a long period of time will eventually cause poisoning. It's interesting that among the "bad" trace minerals, arsenic is not the most potently toxic. In fact the "good" trace mineral fluoride is a much more potent toxin than arsenic and was used as a rat poison before it started being dumped into our municipal water supplies. (See page 21 for a more in-depth discussion of water fluoridation.)

It may also surprise you to know that your body needs arsenic—it is a necessary nutrient—although in extremely small amounts, which you easily get just by eating and drinking. In industrialized countries it's much more likely that you're getting an overdose of arsenic via industrial smokestacks, fungicides, pesticides, herbicides and cigarette smoke.

Excess arsenic can cause high blood pressure; skin abnormalities such as odd pigmentation, lesions and psoriasis; diarrhea; symptoms of heartburn and indigestion; cancer; and poor circulation. There is also some evidence that chronic overexposure to arsenic can be a causative factor in diabetes.

CADMIUM

Our major source of overexposure to the trace mineral cadmium is agricultural dependence on superphosphate fertilizers. Crops grown with them will absorb higher than normal levels of cadmium from the soil. Cadmium is not only toxic in and of itself in small amounts, it also displaces zinc, one of our most essential trace minerals. Cadimium replaces zinc in plants and animals, and is absorbed in greater amounts when zinc is deficient. Thus, like many of the toxic trace minerals, there is a double jeopardy, with overexposure to cadmium causing a deficiency of zinc and the potential for all the resulting illnesses. This is one of the best reasons I can think of to eat organic fruits and vegetables, aside from not being exposed to pesticides.

Cadmium is also an industrial waste product, and can be poisonous in doses as small as three parts per million. Alcoholic drinks like wine and whiskey are relatively high in cadmium, and cigarette smoke is a significant source. In fact, cadmium is probably one of the main sources of illness in those exposed to second-hand smoke. Pregnant women who smoke are more likely to give birth to zinc-deficient babies.

Cadmium also blocks the absorption of iron. In studies on the effects of cadium done with rodents, the immune system was compromised. Overexposure to cadmium also causes lung, kidney and liver disease, high blood pressure, and may play a role in Alzheimer's disease.

LEAD

According to the medical journal *Lancet,* some historians believe that lead contamination in wine decanters and other cookware in ancient Rome lead to its downfall, due to widespread lead poisoning among the upper classes. As farfetched as this theory might sound, it's not implausible, because the effects of lead poisoning are subtle and insidious, and lead to deterioration of the brain.

More recently, prior to the 1970s, lead was widely used in the U.S. in interior house paint. For this reason, lead is still an incredibly common source of poisoning, especially among children. If you live in one of the estimated 40 million houses in the U.S. that still has lead-based paint inside, you, your family and pets may be breathing lead-laden dust. It's more than worth it, if you live in a house built prior to 1976, to have your house dust- or paint-tested for lead.

If you do find that you have high levels of lead in your house paint or dust, it's important to cover it or remove it. If you remove it, be sure to take precautions not to breathe the dust created, or allow your family and pets to breathe it. Small children and pregnant women should not be allowed in a house where leaded paint is being removed. If you have lead paint on the outside of your house, it can wash off the side of the house and into the soil, polluting areas where children play or where pets spend time.

Those children most susceptible to lead poisoning live in urban slums where paint is peeling and there was, prior to the early 1990s when leaded gasoline was finally phased out, excessive lead in the air from car exhaust.

And here's the typical toxic trace mineral double jeopardy: zinc deficiency can exacerbate lead poisoning, and zinc supplementation may prevent it. While those in poverty in the U.S. aren't typically starving, their nutrition tends to be very poor, with an emphasis on refined white flours, chips, soda, sugary foods and other processed foods devoid of the essential trace minerals such as zinc. Children from low-income families have been shown to be deficient in dietary zinc, so not only are they over-exposed to lead, they are deficient in the very mineral that could help them avoid lead poisoning.

But lead doesn't just take up where zinc left off. Where lead is present in high levels, and calcium and magnesium are low, the body will take up lead instead of calcium and magnesium. Sufficient dietary calcium and magnesium can also help prevent lead poisoning.

Premature infants also tend to be deficient in zinc. Lead poisoning in children can cause mental retardation, stunted growth, hearing loss, anemia, high blood pressure, hyperactivity, aggressiveness, kidney disease, poor coordination, learning disabilities, and lower IQ. According to a report published in the *Journal of the American Medical Association*, a study that evaluated 503 first grade children for lead exposure found that higher levels of lead were associated with antisocial and delinquent behavior. When nutrition is very poor and lead exposure very high, even death may result.

Another source of lead is tap water polluted by old plumbing soldered with lead. The EPA (Environmental Protection Agency) estimates that one out of every six households in America have toxic levels of lead in their water. Tin cans soldered with lead used to be a source of lead poisoning in the U.S., and in many countries still are. Children may chew on toys with lead-based paints. Cigarette smoke is a source of lead. Lead crystal decanters, if used to store wine or other alcoholic or acidic beverages, can be a significant source of lead. Even a lead crystal glass filled with wine will leach tiny amounts of lead.

One of the most common sources of lead poisoning among adults in North America is ceramic pots, plates, cups, pitchers, casserole dishes and other cookware and food storage containers bought in foreign countries that don't regulate lead content, such as Mexico,

South America and Asia. If you buy these items outside of North America, I recommend you test them for lead before eating off them or using them to store food.

Symptoms of lead poisoning in adults can include confusion, headaches, constipation, fatigue, weight loss, high blood pressure, kidney disease, degenerative brain diseases, reproductive abnormalities and digestive problems. According to a study done at Harvard Medical School, even low levels of lead poisoning can cause kidney dysfunction in older men. Over-exposure to lead is also associated with cancer, probably because lead interferes with the production of glutathione, your body's first level of antioxidant defense.

MERCURY

The single biggest source of exposure to the toxic trace mineral mercury is dental fillings called amalgams, which contain a mix of metals, including mercury. Because mercury is a liquid metal at room temperature, and changes easily with changes in temperature and pressure, it readily gives off fumes which are inhaled by those with amalgam fillings.

Unfortunately, the toxicity of mercury fillings is not acknowledged by the American Dental Association, presumably due to fear of billions of dollars in class action lawsuits if they admit to the dangers of this extremely toxic and volatile heavy metal. In other countries mercury amalgams have been well studied, and it is clear that the more mercury amalgam fillings a person has, the higher the mercury concentrations in their blood and urine. Both dentists and dental assistants frequently show symptoms of mercury poisoning. Germany and Sweden have banned the use of mercury in dental fillings.

I strongly recommend that you not have any new

mercury amalgams put in, and if you are suffering from symptoms of mercury poisoning, have them taken out and replaced with porcelain fillings. (Gold fillings can contain high levels of cadmium.) There is no perfect substance to use for filling cavities in teeth, but porcelain seems to be the most benign right now.

Mercury is yet another heavy metal that is a common by-product of industrial wastes, and it is also a common waste product in hospitals. It is often dumped into waterways or the ocean, where it is ingested by shellfish and fish. Large fish that live near coastlines often have very high levels of mercury in their flesh. Swordfish and large tuna have the highest levels of mercury.

Mercury is one of the most toxic of the heavy metals, as it inhibits the body's use of the important B vitamin folic acid, and alters protein structures, which are involved in every aspect of bodily function.

Symptoms of mercury poisoning can include birth defects in the children of mothers exposed to it in utero, and central nervous system damage such as is seen in multiple sclerosis and Alzheimer's disease. Other symptoms include insomnia, anorexia, chronic fatigue, depression, headaches, diarrhea, irregular heartbeat, hair loss, irritability, kidney damage, loss of sex drive and muscle weakness. Mercury suppresses the immune system and creates a high susceptibility to infection.

If you break a thermometer in your home and spill mercury, cleaning it up can cause signficant amounts of mercury to escape into the air, carpets and dust of the house. Pregnant women and small children should be removed from the room for at least 24 hours, and the mercury should be carefully scooped up and placed in a closed glass container. The container should be disposed of at a hazardous waste facility. Then the area where the mercury spilled should be carefully vacuumed up, and the bag immediately disposed of.

NICKEL

Nickel is a trace mineral that is needed for the maintenance of health in very small amounts, but can quickly become toxic. Nickel is found in our RNA, and is thought to play a role in enzyme function. Overexposure to nickel can cause heart disease, cancer, skin disorders and thyroid malfunction. Since nickel is not a commonly used metal, overexposure to it is rare.

TIN

Poisoning from tin used to be a major health problem due to canning and storage of food in tin containers with no inner coating, but today it is rare. Caution should be used when eating canned foods outside North America. Some processed foods may contain tin-based preservatives and stabilizers.

Overexposure to tin may interfere with the body's production of glutathione, an important antioxidant, and block the absorption of copper, zinc and iron.

CHELATION THERAPY AND OTHER DETOXIFIERS

Mainstream medicine is largely at a loss to effectively handle heavy metal poisoning, but for years alternative doctors and other health-care professionals have sucessfully used chelation therapy to rid the body of these toxins and also to treat heart disease. Chelation therapy is controversial largely because it competes with prescription drugs and is a safe and effective alternative to them. Opponents claim that EDTA (ethylene diamine tetraacetic acid), the synthetic amino acid used in chelation, can produce kidney damage, but this is caused by factors such as dosage and biochemistry that are now taken into account, and there hasn't been an instance of kidney damage with EDTA use since the early 1960s.

Chelation therapy uses EDTA or other chelating agents, given intravenously over a period of many weeks or months in 20-30 treatments. At the same time, essential vitamins and minerals are given. EDTA essentially latches onto heavy metals that have accumulated in the tissues, combining with them to form compounds that can be excreted from the body. Chelation therapy is well studied, and has been used in at least half a million people. Remarkable results have been achieved using it for children with lead poisoning, and in adults with heart disease, Alzheimer's disease and arthritis.

Substances found in seaweed called alginates have been found to bind with some heavy metals, including strontium, cadmium, barium, radium and lead. Regularly adding dried seaweed products to meals can be a kind of health insurance against heavy metal poisoning.

Saunas and sweat baths are said to sweat out heavy metals, but this is hard on the body if you are already weakened by toxins.

One of the best allies against the accumulation of heavy metals in the body is proper nutrition. Getting plenty of the "good" trace minerals and enough of the body's other needed nutrients for optimal health will give your body the armament it needs to fight heavy metals.

GLOSSARY

absorption The process by which nutrients are passed into the bloodstream.

alkaline Containing an acid-neutralizing substance (being alkaline, sodium bicarbonate is used for excess acidity in foods).

amino acid chelates Chelated minerals that have been produced by many of the same processes nature uses to chelate minerals in the body; in the digestive tract, nature surrounds the elemental minerals with amino acid, permitting them to be absorbed into the bloodstream.

amino acids The organic compounds from which proteins are constructed; 22 amino acids have been identified as necessary to the human body; nine are known as essential—histidine, isoleucine, leucine, lysine, total S-containing amino acids, total aromatic amino acids, threonine, tryptophan, and valine—and must be obtained from food.

anorexia Abnormal fear of becoming obese, a persistent aversion to food, a distorted self-image, and severe loss of weight.

antioxidant A substance that can protect another substance from oxidation; added to foods to keep oxygen from changing the food's color.

arthritis Inflammation of joints.

arteriosclerosis A disease of the arteries characterized by hardening, thickening, and loss of elasticity of the arterial walls; results in impaired blood circulation.

assimilation The process whereby nutrients are used by the body and changed into living tissue.

asthma A condition of lungs characterized by a decrease in diameter of some air passages; a spasm of the bronchial tubes or swelling of their mucous membranes.

atherosclerosis A process whereby fatty deposits in the walls of arteries make the walls thick and hard, narrowing the arteries; a form of arteriosclerosis.

autoimmunity An abnormal condition whereby the body produces antibodies against its own tissues.

beta-carotene A plant pigment which can be converted into two forms of vitamin A.

carcinogen A cancer-causing substance.

cardiovascular Relating to the heart and blood vessels.

carotene An orange-yellow pigment occurring in many plants and capable of being converted into vitamin A in the body.

catalyst A substance that modifies, especially increases, the rate of chemical reaction without being consumed or changed in the process.

chelation A process by which mineral substances are changed into an easily digestible form.

cholesterol A white, crystalline substance, made up of various fats; naturally produced in vertebrate animals and humans; important as a precursor to steroid hormones and as a constituent of cell membranes.

coenzyme A substance that combines with other substances to form a complete enzyme; nonprotein and usually a B vitamin.

collagen The primary organic constituent of bone,

cartilage and connective tissue (becomes gelatin through boiling).

demineralization The loss of minerals or salts from bone and tissue.

diuretic Tending to increase the flow of urine from the body.

endocrine Producing secretions passed directly to the lymph or blood instead of into a duct; to do with the endocrine glands or the hormones they produce.

enzyme A protein substance found in living cells that brings about chemical changes; necessary for digestion of food; compounds with names ending in -ase.

FDA Food and Drug Administration.

gland An organ in the body where certain substances in the blood are separated and converted into secretions for use in the body (such as hormones) or to be discharged from the body (such as sweat); nonsecreting structures similar to glands, like lymph nodes, are also known as glands.

glucose Blood sugar; a product of the body's assimilation of carbohydrates and a major source of energy.

HDL High-density lipoprotein; HDL is sometimes called "good" cholesterol because it is the body's major carrier of cholesterol to the liver for excretion in the bile.

hemoglobin Molecule necessary for the transport of oxygen by red blood cells; iron is an essential component.

homeostasis The body's physiological equilibrium.

hormone A substance formed in endocrine organs and transported by body fluids to activate other specifically receptive organs, cells or tissues.

hydrochloric acid An acid secreted in the stomach; a main part of gastric juice.

immune Protected against disease.

insulin A hormone, secreted by the pancreas, that helps regulate the metabolism of sugar in the body.

LDL Low-density lipoprotein; sometimes referred to as "bad" cholesterol, LDLs easily become oxidized and carry cholesterol through the bloodstream; studies show high levels can increase risk of coronary artery disease (CAD).

metabolism The processes of physical and chemical change whereby food is synthesized into living matter until it is broken down into simpler substances or waste matter; energy is produced by these processes.

organic Describes any chemical containing carbon; or any food or supplement made with animal or vegetable fertilizers; or produced without synthetic fertilizers or pesticides and free from chemical injections or additives.

oxalates Organic chemicals found in certain foods, especially spinach, which can combine with calcium to form calcium oxalate, an insoluble chemical the body cannot use.

oxidation The way in which certain types of altered oxygen molecules cause biochemical reactions; examples are browning of apples and rancidity in oil.

protein A complex substance containing nitrogen which is essential to plant and animal cells; ingested proteins are changed to amino acids in the body.

RDA Recommended Dietary Allowances as established by the Food and Nutrition Board, National Academy of Sciences, National Research Council.

T-Cells White blood cells, manufactured in the thymus, which protect the body from bacteria, viruses, and cancer-causing agents, while controlling the production of B-cells which produce antibodies, and unwanted production of potentially harmful T-cells.

toxicity The quality or condition of being poisonous, harmful, or destructive.

toxin An organic poison produced in living or dead organisms.

triglycerides Fatty substances in the blood.

USRDA United States Recommended Daily Allowances.

vitamin Any of about fifteen natural compounds essential in small amounts as catalysts for processes in the body; most cannot be made by the body and must come from diet.

BIBLIOGRAPHY

Bigazzi, Pierluigi E., "Autoimmunity and Heavy Metals," *Lupus*, 1994;3:449-453.

DiCyan, E., *A Beginner's Introduction to Trace Minerals*, Keats Publishing, New Canaan, Conn., 1984

Earth Matters, issue # 30, Friends of the Earth, London, Summer 1996.

Hauser, Robert, A., et al., "Blood Manganese Correlates with Brain Magnetic Resonance Imaging Changes in Patients with Liver Disease," *Canadian Journal of Neurological Science*, May 1996;23(2):95-98.

Hendler, S., *The Doctor's Vitamin and Mineral Encyclopedia*, Fireside, NY, 1991.

Hu, Howard, M.D., ScD., et al., "The Relationship of Bone and Blood Lead to Hypertension: The Normative Aging Study," *JAMA*, April 17, 1996;275-(15):1171-1176.

Jensen, B., et al., *Empty Harvest*, Avery Publishing Group Inc., Garden City Park, N.Y., 1990.

Kim, Rokho, M.D., Dr.P.H., et al., "A Longitudinal Study of Low-Level Lead Exposure and Impairment of Renal Function, The Normative Aging Study" *JAMA*, April 17, 1996;275(15):1177-1181.

Laino, Charlene, "City Air Pollution Linked to Male Infertility," *Medical Tribune*, November 9, 1995;14.

Martlew, G., *Electrolytes, the Spark of Life*, Nature's Publishing, Ltd., Murdock, Fla., 1994.

McClanahan, Mark, A., "Mercury Contamination in the Home," *The Lancet*, April 13, 1996;347:1044-1045.

Mesch, U., et al., "Lead Poisoning Masquerading as Chronic Fatigue Syndrome," *The Lancet*, April 27, 1996;347:1193.

Needleman, Herbert, L., et al., "Bone Lead Levels and Delinquent Behavior," *JAMA*, February 7, 1996;275(5):363-369.

Rader J.I., "Anti-nutritive Effects of Dietary Tin," *Adv. Exp. Med. Biol.*, 1991; 289:509-24.

Rahman, Mahfuzar and Axelson, Olav, "Diabetes Mellitus and Arsenic Exposure: A Second Look at Case-Control Data From a Swedish Copper Smelter," *Occupational and Environmental Medicine*, 1995;52:773-774.

Schmitt, Nicholas, "Could Zinc Help Protect Children From Lead Poisoning," *Canadian Medical Association Journal*, January 1, 1996;154(1):13-14.

Schroeder, H., *The Trace Elements and Man*, Devin-Adair, Greenwich, Conn., 1973

Sehnert, K.W., Clague, A.F. and Cheraskin, E., "Improvement in Renal Function Following EDTA Chelation and Multi-Vitamin-Trace Mineral Therapy: A Study in Creatinine Clearance," *Med. Hypotheses*, Nov 1984;15(3):301-4.

Somer, E., *The Essential Guide to Vitamins and Minerals*, HarperCollins, New York, 1995.

Stadtler, Von P., "Amalgam," *Occupation and Environment*, 1995;43:163-171.

Vaughn, L. et al., *Prevention Magazine's Complete Book of Vitamins and Minerals*," Wings Books, Avenel, N.J., 1994.

INDEX